Beauty Face Mask

From Home

Vevine Goldson

Beauty Face Mask

Face Spa Right From Home

ISBN-13:978-1976585708

ISBN-10:1976585708

Dedication

This book is written for anyone that wants to achieve a flawless complexion without going to a spa. Others just want to go the organic way and there are a lot of creative Beauty Uses for common staples. You don't have to go to a spa to find the best skincare face masks to achieve a perfect and flawless skin. You will find Spa from home in this book face mask that can match any beauty spots.

Contents

1. Honey mayonnaise and goat milk powder
2. Banana lemon and honey mask
3. Strawberry yogurt and honey mask
4. Cornmeal honey and egg yolk
5. Lemon Oatmeal and mayonnaise
6. Powdered goats milk and pure orange juice
7. Avocado cucumber and olive oil
8. Mayonnaise strawberry and oatmeal
9. Turmeric yogurt and coconut oil
10. Avocado honey and brown sugar
11. Coconut oil goats milk and oatmeal
12. Blueberries olive oil and honey
13. Orange juice mayonnaise and coconut oil
14. Sugar Olive Oil and yogurt
15. Orange Juice lemon and honey mask
16. Banana coconut oil and yogurt
17. Lemons apple and buttermilk
18. Tomato yogurt and olive oil
19. Buttermilk oatmeal and coconut oil
20. Aloe Vera gel honey and lemon
21. Avocado tomato and mayonnaise
22. Apple cedar vinegar coconut and yogurt
23. Avocado Turmeric and castor oil
24. Blueberries banana and lemon juice
25. Goats milk strawberries castor oil and oatmeal
26. Kiwi fruit oatmeal and castor oil
27. Yogurt kiwi fruit and milk powder
28. Aloe Vera gel turmeric and mayonnaise honey
29. Pumpkin oatmeal honey yogurt
30. Melon honey egg white cornmeal yogurt

Introduction

Why these masks are good? They calm the skin and provide vitamins anti-oxidants

and minerals; they help to repair damaged skin tissues, They tighten pores, make fine lines less Visible, removes dead skin cells revealing softer more supple skin. These masks will leave you with a healthy glow! You don't have to go to a spa to find the best skincare masks to achieve a perfect and flawless skin.

> Making your own homemade beauty face masks is relatively simple. I share my most popular 30 recipes that will be beneficial to the skin all from natural ingredients. You'll be able to find these ingredients for the recipes in your kitchen.

I have been using these treatments for a long time and years ago I use to give my friends a beauty facial for their birthdays using these same kitchen staples and they were amazed at how good they work. These mask are extremely recommended because they are made from all natural products which in turn provide essential and well needed nutrients to the skin. Effort will yield good results.

Honey mayonnaise and goats milk powder

Honey is natural anti-bacterial syrup which is great for treating acne and removes dryness while slowing down aging and mayonnaise is packed with ingredients that can help to nourish your skin. This honey-and-mayonnaise with goat milk powder will leave your face with an organic and healthy glow. Goat's milk is packed with vitamin A and E that promotes clear and beautiful skin.

Here is how to make it.

1. Add two tea spoons full of powdered goat milk

2. one large spoon full of mayonnaise

3. and one large spoon full of honey

 in a container then Mix into a smooth paste.

You can thicken or weaken your mask by adding a

bit of warm water or adding more of an ingredient.

Apply to washed clean face for 30 minutes then wash off the face mask with cool or Luke warm water or warm face cloth. Pat face dry enjoy your beautiful glowing skin!

Banana lemon and honey mask

Designed for all skin types this mask will leave skin supple beautiful and hydrated. Honey is antibacterial and soothing, and lemon juice is a natural skin brightener that eliminates black heads and help to fade discolorations. Bananas have minerals and vitamins that are known to tighten pores shrink acne while leaving skin hydrated and well moisturized.

1. Mash half of a ripe banana into a container.

2. Add one tablespoon of lemon juice and and one table spoon of organic honey.

Mix the ingredients together. You can thicken or weaken your mask by adding a

bit of warm water or adding more of an ingredient.

3. Apply to clean washed face for 30 minutes then wash

off the face mask with cool or Luke warm water. You can

also remove face masks with a warm face cloth

Pat face dry enjoy a rejuvenated and healthy glows!

Strawberry yogurt and honey

This mask will tone your skin and improve the skin's texture, Yogurt improves the skin's elastin and will leave it bright and clear and helps to improve dark circles. Strawberries are power packed with Vitamin C which helps to boost the production of collagen minimises fine lines and wrinkles. Ancient Romans use to use strawberries to beautify their skin. The honey will rehydrate and moisturize penetrate deeply into the skin's surface leaving it with a beautiful glow.

1.Crush two soft strawberries in a container

2.add one spoon full of plain yogurt

3.add one spoon full of organic honey

You can thicken or weaken your mask by adding a

bit of warm water or adding more of an ingredient.

mix the three ingredients together and apply to clean washed face.

Leave on for 15 to 30 minutes before wash leave mine on for 30 minutes.

Remove with Luke warm water or warm face cloth.

Enjoy revitalized and glowing skin!

Cornmeal honey and egg yolk

This facial both exfoliates and moisturizes. Cornmeal contains zinc manganese iron and copper and traces minerals. When mixed with other kitchen staples will make an excellent face mask and gentle enough so it will not irritate the skin. The honey helps prevent aging giving skin a more youthful glow and eggs are loaded with proteins and fats that are good for the skin when applied topically, egg yolk is known to help moisturise and heal dry skin.

1.Add one large spoon full of cornmeal

2.Two tablespoons of organic honey

3.The yolk of an egg

You can thicken or weaken your mask by adding a

bit of warm water or adding more of an ingredient.

Mix well together until the ingredients are all blended smoothly. Wash dirt and makeup from face then apply the face mask gently rubbing in circular motion. After 18-30 minutes wash face with Luke warm water. Pat dry enjoy glowing healthy skin!

Lemon Oatmeal and mayonnaise

Egg white is commonly known to be effective in tightening skin, and the proteins from the eggs contain in the mayonnaise helps to provide nourishment for the skin. Oatmeal contains salicylic acid which has exfoliating properties. Lemons are rich in citric acid and Vitamin C brighten dull skin and act as an astringent that removes white heads black heads and shrink acne.

1. Add two table spoon of lemon

2. Add two large spoonsful of oatmeal

3. Add two large spoon of mayonnaise

You can thicken or weaken your mask by adding a

bit of warm water or adding more of an ingredient.

Pour a little bit of warm water in Whip them together until they become frothy and blend to form a paste. Wash makeup Clean from face then apply the ingredients for 15 to 30 minutes.

Wash with Luke warm water or remove with a warm wash cloth. Pat face dry, enjoy nice beautiful

glowing supple skin!

Powdered goats milk and pure orange juice

Orange is power packed with vitamin c and antioxidants. The strong antioxidants in this sweet fruit are known to combat free radicals and when applied topically can be used to treat acne prone skin, and lighten hyper pigmented areas. Goats milk has healing properties that is good for skin and the lactic acid found in it helps to exfoliate and soften the skin leaving it with a supple texture.

Rejuvenate your skin with this simple mask.

1.Mix 1/4 cup powdered milk with enough water to form a thick paste

2. Add two large spoonsful of organic orange juice and

   Mix in well.

You can thicken or weaken your mask by adding a

bit of warm water or adding more of an ingredient.

Wash face of any dirt and impurities then apply evenly

 leave mask on for 15 to 30 minutes. Remove with Luke warm water or warm face cloth.

Enjoy clean smooth soft and beautiful skin!

Avocado cucumber and olive oil

The avocado with its fleshy green pulp contains fibre vitamins minerals such as vitamin k, and is extremely hydrating, Due to its many nutrients it is effective in treating damaged skin and is a good moisturizer when applied topically. Cucumbers are rich in water and contain insoluble fibre. Cucumber is known to treat freckles tighten pores tones and cool inflamed skin. Olive oil contains powerful antioxidants and is anti-inflammatory oil.

1 Add 1/2 a small avocado in a dish

2. Add two large spoons full off cucumber juice

3. Add one large spoon full of virgin olive oil

You can thicken or weaken your mask by adding a

bit of warm water or adding more of an ingredient.

Crush and mix well until everything is smoothly pasted together. Wash face clean and apply for 15 to 30 minutes wash with Luke warm water. Enjoy a beautiful well moisturized and glowing skin!

Mayonnaise strawberry and oatmeal

The Omega- 3 fatty acids found in strawberries lighten the skin tone and reduce dark circles, and help to get rid of of dead skin cells. Oatmeal contains salicylic acid which has exfoliating properties, it gently remove impurities from blocked pores and is an excellent remedy to treat dry skin. Traditional mayonnaise is made with whole eggs and vinegar so Mayonnaise is a high source of protein and protein is really good for skin when applied topically. Here is how to make this mask.

1.Add 1/4 cup size some oatmeal in a container, pour warm water and mix into a creamy paste.

2. Add the puree of three ripe strawberries to the mixture.

3. Add two large spoonsful of mayonnaise.

You can thicken or weaken your mask by adding a

bit of warm water or adding more of an ingredient.

Mix together well until everything is blended in.

Wash face clean and apply mask for 15-30 minutes.

Remove with Luke warm water or warm face cloth.

Enjoy beautiful soft clear skin!

Turmeric yogurt and coconut oil

This edible food source Turmeric is great for skin and has been used as a medicinal agent in Chinese and siddha practices for many years. Turmeric is extremely good for the skin because of its anti-inflammatory and anti-bacterial practices. Yogurt improves the skin's elastin and will leave it bright and clear and helps to improve dark circles. Coconut oil contains anti-fungal properties, remove dead skin cells and the oil does not clog pores.

Here is how to make this mask

1.Add one tea spoonful of turmeric in a container

2.Add one teaspoonful of organic coconut oil

3.Add two large spoonsful of plain yogurt

You can thicken or weaken your mask by adding a

bit of warm water or adding more of an ingredient.

Mix together until smoothly blend. Wash face clean

removing any traces of makeup then apply mask on

dry clean face.

Keep on for 15 to 30 minutes then wash off with

luke warm water or warm face cloth. If you find that the

turmeric stains the face wipe face with cotton bud

dipped in facial toner or warm water.

Enjoy beautiful soft rejuvenated clear skin!

Avocado honey and brown sugar

Apply this mask before an event as it gets your skin soft and glowing. Sugar is a natural source of glycolic acid and is very easy to work with. It is very effective in the treatment of sun-damaged and aging skin. When add with other ingredients makes an excellent scrub and removes roughness from elbows and heels. Honey is a very good skin repairer and makes a perfect base for any mask. Avocado has vitamin E B and C which is excellent for any skin.

1.Add 1/2 of a small avocado into a container

2.Add two teaspoonful of organic honey

3.Add one and a half large spoon of brown sugar.

Crush blend and mix together until smooth.

 You can thicken or weaken your mask by adding a

bit of warm water or adding more of an ingredient.

Wash face removing any traces of makeup and other

Moisturizer then apply this mask for 15-30

Minutes. Remove with warm face cloth or wash

with Luke warm water. Enjoy clear glowing soft skin!

Coconut oil goat's milk and oatmeal

Coconut oil is rich in saturated fats that is provide excellent benefits to skin when used as a topical

Treatment. Goat milk is rich in calcium and lots of mineral and has healing properties when applied to skin, and has antifungal properties. Oatmeal contains salicylic acid which has exfoliating properties, it gently remove impurities from blocked pores and is an excellent remedy to treat dry skin.

1.Add quarter cup oatmeal in a container

2. Add pour just enough goat milk in it and mix into a paste.

3. Add one teaspoon full of organic coconut oil. Stir and mix the ingredients together.

You can thicken or weaken your mask by adding a

bit of warm water or adding more of an ingredient.

Wash dirt and makeup from face pat dry then apply mask. Let it stay for 15 to 30 minutes.

Wash with Luke warm water or remove with a warm wash cloth. You will see and feel the difference on your skin!

Blueberries olive oil and honey

Blueberries are rich in Vitamin C and anti-oxidants, contain a good amount of other nutrients which can boost collagen. Olive oil contains powerful antioxidants and is calming to the skin when used as a topical treatment. The honey helps prevent aging giving skin a more youthful glow is a very good skin repairer and makes a perfect base for any mask and Will help to hydrate the skin leaving it soft and glowing.

1.Add a five to six blueberries in a container

2.Add one teaspoonful of virgin olive oil

3.Add one large spoonful of organic honey

Crush and mix the ingredients together until they blend smoothly in a paste.

You can thicken or weaken your mask by adding a

bit of warm water or adding more of an ingredient.

Wash face of any traces of makeup and dirt then apply generous amount on

your face, massage in. Let it stay 15 to 30 minutes.

Wash face with Luke warm water or warm wash cloth. Your skin will have a youthful

 and supple look enjoy!

Orange juice mayonnaise and coconut oil

Orange has a lot of vitamin c and is a very powerful and strong anti-oxidant which is great for treating acne prone skin and blackheads. Mayonnaise is a high source of protein and protein is really good for skin when applied topically is good for the hair and skin. Coconut oil has antimicrobial properties that can help to fight bacteria and is used as an important

Ingredient in several skin creams.

1. Add two large spoonsful of mayonnaise in a container

2.Add one large spoonful of organic orange juice

3. Add one teaspoonful of organic coconut oil.

Mix the ingredients together until equally blend.

You can thicken or weaken your mask by adding a

bit of warm water or adding more of an ingredient.

Wash face of makeup and old moisture pat dry and

Keep on for 15 to 30 minutes. Wash with Luke warm water or wipe with warm face cloth.

Enjoy soft clear beautiful skin!

14

Sugar Olive Oil and yogurt

Sugar is a natural source of glycolic acid and is one of the best home stables that helps to exfoliate the skin removing dead cells. Olive oil contains powerful antioxidants and is calming to the skin.

Yogurt especially the plain yogurt is a good skin repairer, when used topically it repairs the skins elastin leaving it with a clear youthful glow.

1.Add half cup virgin olive oil in a container

2.Add half cup brown sugar

Mix the ingredients together and place in a jar.

You can thicken or weaken your mask by adding a

bit of warm water or adding more of an ingredient.

Store in a fridge and whenever you are ready you can use it as a face scrub.

To use this as a face mask scoop two teaspoons full of it and mix it with a large spoon full of yogurt. Remember to wash face first before applying. Let it stay for 15 to 30 minutes then wash off with Luke warm water or warm face cloth. Enjoy a soft and beautiful well hydrated skin!

Orange Juice lemon and honey

Give yourself a TLC without wandering too far, this one is really easy to make.

Orange and lemons are high in vitamin c and certain types of acid that exfoliates and

brighten dull and acne prone skin. Helps in removing unsightly and uneven tan and lightens pigmentation marks on sun damaged skin. The honey with its many skin healing properties penetrates deep into the skins epidermis and helps to soften and make fine lines less visible.

1.Add one large spoonful of orange juice

2.Add one teaspoonful of lemon

3.Add one teaspoonful of organic honey.

You can thicken or weaken your mask by adding a

bit of warm water or adding more of an ingredient.

Mix the ingredients together until equally blend. Wash face of makeup and old moisture pat dry and keep on for 15 to 30 minutes. wash with Luke warm water or wipe with warm face cloth.

Enjoy soft clear beautiful skin!

Banana coconut oil and yogurt

Bananas have minerals and vitamins that are known to tighten pores shrink acne while leaving skin hydrated and well moisturized. Coconut oil is rich in saturated fats that is provide Excellent benefits to skin and help remove dead skin cells. Yogurt improves the skin's elastin and will leave it bright and clear and helps to improve dark circles while improving the skins texture as it heals and tones.

1.Add half banana in a container

2.Add one teaspoonful of organic coconut oil

3.Add two teaspoons full of yogurt

Crush and mix the ingredients together until they are smoothly blend.

You can thicken or weaken your mask by adding a

bit of warm water or adding more of an ingredient.

Wash face of makeup and old moisture pat dry and

keep on for 15 to 30 minutes.

wash with Luke warm water or wipe with warm face cloth.

Enjoy soft clear beautiful skin!

Lemon apple and buttermilk

Apples are power packed with vitamins and other natural ingredients that will make any skin glow.

Lemons are rich in citric acid and Vitamin C brighten dull skin and act as an astringent that removes white heads black heads and shrink acne. Buttermilk is a very effective treatment that contains lactic acid which helps to reduce fine lines and wrinkles while softening and repairing.

1.chop up one green apple

2.Add half cup of butter milk

3.Add one large spoonful of lemon

Blend crush and mix until you get a smooth paste.

You can thicken or weaken your mask by adding a

bit of warm water or adding more of an ingredient.

Apply to clean washed face for 30 minutes then wash

off the face mask with cool or Luke warm water. You can

 also remove face masks with a warm face cloth

 Pat face dry enjoy a rejuvenated and healthy glows!

Tomato yogurt and olive oil

Tomatoes are packed with lots of nutrients and anti-oxidants that are good for skin. It is rich in vitamin A C and folic acid. It repairs and is especially good for acne neutralizes free radicals and balances the ph. zone. Yogurt improves the skin's elastin and will leave it bright and clear and helps to improve dark circles. Olive oil contains powerful antioxidants and is calming to the skin balances the skin while moisturizing it.

1.chop up one tomato

2.Add quarter cup yogurt

3.Add two spoonsful of virgin olive oil

Blend together until it is smooth.

You can thicken or weaken your mask by adding a

bit of warm water or adding more of an ingredient.

Wash face of any dirt and impurities then apply evenly

leave mask on for 15 to 30 minutes.

Remove with Luke warm water or warm face cloth.

Enjoy clean smooth soft and beautiful skin!

Buttermilk oatmeal and coconut oil

Oatmeal contains salicylic acid which has exfoliating agents, it gently remove impurities from blocked pores and is an excellent remedy to treat dry skin. Buttermilk is a very effective treatment that contains lactic acid which helps to reduce fine lines and wrinkles while it cleanses. Coconut oil is rich in saturated fats that are provide excellent benefits to skin and help remove dead skin from the surface cells.

1.Add half cup of oats in a container, pour some warm water in and make a smooth paste.

2.Add one large spoon- full of butter milk

3.Add one teaspoonful of organic coconut oil

Mix everything together.

You can thicken or weaken your mask by adding a

bit of warm water or adding more of an ingredient.

Wash face removing any traces of makeup and other

Moisturizer then applies this mask for 15-30 minutes.

Remove with warm face cloth or wash

with Luke warm water. Enjoy clear glowing soft skin!

Aloe Vera gel honey and lemon

Aloe Vera is a great item for treating sun burnt skin because of its natural anti-inflammatory agents. It calms irritation and help in the relief of discomfort, repairs dry skin while it moisturizes and rejuvenates the skin. Lemon juice is a natural skin brightener that eliminates black heads and help to fade discolorations. Honey is a natural anti-bacterial syrup which is great for treating acne and helps to slow down the aging process.

1.Add two spoonsful of aloe Vera gel

2.Add one spoonful of organic honey

3.Add one spoonful of lemon

Mix the two ingredients together until they

it is equally mixed.

You can thicken or weaken your mask by adding a

bit of warm water or adding more of an ingredient.

Wash makeup Clean from face then apply the ingredients for 15 to 30 minutes.

Wash with Luke warm water or remove with a warm wash cloth. Pat face dry, enjoy nice beautiful

glowing supple skin!

Avocado tomato and mayonnaise

Avocado is extremely hydrating. Avocados green pulpy flesh is very effective to treat and repair skin because it is packed with nutrients that rehydrates while it moisturizes. avocado has vitamin E B and C which is excellent for any skin. Traditional mayonnaise is made with whole eggs and vinegar so Mayonnaise is a high source of protein and protein is really good for skin when applied topically. Tomatoes has anti-oxidants that are good for skin, It is rich in vitamin A C and folic acid.

1.Add half of a small avocado in a container

2.Add one table spoon of tomato puree

3.Add one large spoon of mayonnaise

Mix together until everything is smoothly blend.

You can thicken or weaken your mask by adding a

bit of warm water or adding more of an ingredient.

Wash face clean and apply mask for 15-30 minutes.

Remove with Luke warm water or warm face cloth. You'll love your new fresh face enjoy!

Apple cedar vinegar coconut and yogurt

Apple Cider Vinegar contains AHA that can de-clog blocked pores and remove dead cells from the skin's surface. It is a good treatment for acne prone skin. Yogurt improves the skin's elastin and will leave it bright and clear and helps to improve dark circles.

Coconut oil is rich in healthy fats that provide excellent benefits to skin and help remove dead skin cells.

1.Add one large spoonful of apple cedar vinegar

2.Add one teaspoon full of coconut oil

3.Add two large spoonsful of plain yogurt

Mix the ingredients well together until smoothly blend.

You can thicken or weaken your mask by adding a

bit of warm water or adding more of an ingredient.

removing any traces of makeup then apply mask on

dry clean face. Keep on for 15 to 30 minutes then wash off with

Luke warm water or warm face cloth.

Enjoy soft clear beautiful skin!

Avocado Turmeric and castor oil

Castor oil is rich in omega 3-6-9 fatty acids anti-fungal and antibacterial and has a lot of natural skin healing properties. It helps to slow down aging and make spots appear less visible.

Avocado has vitamin E B and C which is excellent for any skin.

Turmeric is extremely good for the skin because of its anti-inflammatory and anti-bacterial practices.

1.Add half avocado to a container

2.Add one teas poon full of turmeric

3.Add one teaspoon full of organic castor oil

Mix everything together in a paste.

You can thicken or weaken your mask by adding a

bit of warm water or adding more of an ingredient.

Wash face clean and apply for 15 to 30 minutes

Wash with Luke warm water. Enjoy a beautiful well moisturized and

Glowing skin!

Blueberries banana and lemon juice

This mask is extremely good for those that suffer from combination skin. Blueberries are rich in Vitamin C and contain a good amount of anthocyanin, which can boost collagen levels in the skin. Avocado is extremely hydrating. And avocado has vitamin E B and C which is excellent for any skin.

Lemons are rich in citric acid and Vitamin C brighten dull skin and act as an astringent for

acne prone skin and helps to shrink pimples and de-clogs pores.

1.Chop up half a banana in a container

2.Add a small handful of blueberries

3.Add and one teaspoon of lemon juice

Mix crush together until smoothly blend.

You can thicken or weaken your mask by adding a

bit of warm water or adding more of an ingredient.

Apply to clean washed face for 30 minutes then wash   off the face mask with cool or Luke warm water. You can also remove face masks with a warm face cloth

Pat face dry enjoy a rejuvenated and healthy glows!

Goats milk strawberries castor oil and oatmeal

Cleopatra use to use goats milk as a beauty treatment and it is well known that she did have the most flawless and beautiful skin than any women in history.

Omega-3 fatty acids found in strawberries lighten the skin tone and reduce dark circles.

Castor oil is also rich in omega 3-6-9 fatty acids, it helps to heal and repair damage skin.

Goat milk softens and exfoliate dry skin.

1.Add quarter cup goat milk in a container

2.crush and Add three strawberries

3.one teaspoon of organic castor oil

4.Add two large spoonsful of oatmeal

Blend and Mix together until i You can thicken or weaken your mask by adding a

bit of warm water or adding more of an ingredient.t is in a paste.

Wash dirt and makeup from face then apply the

face mask gently rubbing in circular motion. After 18-30 minutes wash face with Luke warm water. Pat dry enjoy glowing healthy skin!

Kiwi fruit oatmeal and castor oil honey

Like strawberries oranges and blueberries the kiwi fruit is power packed with vitamins and

other essential nutrients that is extremely beneficial to the skin.

Oatmeal contains salicylic acid which has exfoliating properties, it gently remove impurities from blocked pores and is an excellent remedy to treat dry skin.

Castor oil is rich in omega 3-6-9 fatty acids anti-fungal and antibacterial and has a lot of natural skin healing properties. Honey is moisturizing and is a great skin rejuvenator.

1.Peel one ripe kiwi fruit

2.Add quarter cup oatmeal in a blender

3.add two teaspoonful's of organic castor oil

4.one large spoon honey

add a little bit of warm water to blend it in a paste then apply to clean washed face.

You can thicken or weaken your mask by adding a

bit of warm water or adding more of an ingredient.

Leave on for 15 to 30 minutes before wash; I leave mine on for 30 minutes. Remove with Luke warm water or warm face cloth. Enjoy revitalized and glowing skin!

Yogurt kiwi fruit and milk powder

The pulp of the kiwi fruit is packed with anti-oxidants and lots of different nutrients, that help to restore and stimulate collagen in the skin.

Milk has healing properties that is good for skin and the lactic acid found in it helps to exfoliate and soften the skin leaving it with a supple texture.

Yogurt improves the skin's elastin and will leave it bright and clear and supple.

1.Quarter cup of milk powder in a container

2.Peel one fully ripen kiwi fruit slice up and add in

3.add quarter cup of yogurt

Mix blend or crush until it is in a past.

You can thicken or weaken your mask by adding a

bit of warm water or adding more of an ingredient.

Wash face clean and apply mask for 15-30 minutes.

Remove with Luke warm water or warm face cloth.

Enjoy beautiful soft clear skin!

Aloe Vera gel turmeric and mayonnaise

Turmeric has been used in many skin healing clinics because of its anti-inflammatory and anti-bacterial agents which helps to speed up the recovery process.

Mayonnaise is packed with protein and other ingredients that can help to nourish your skin. Aloe Vera helps to repair and sooth irritation and inflamed skin, and also help to dry skin while it moisturizes and rejuvenates the skin.

1.Add one teaspoonful of turmeric

2.Add two teaspoons full of aloe Vera gel

3.Add two large spoonsful of mayonnaise

Mix together until the ingredients are equally blend.

You can thicken or weaken your mask by adding a

bit of warm water or adding more of an ingredient.

Apply to washed clean face for 30 minutes then wash

off the face mask with cool or Luke warm water or warm face cloth.

Pat face dry enjoy your radiant glowing skin!

Pumpkin oatmeal honey yogurt

This facial beautify exfoliates soothes and moisturizes. While we are getting ready for Halloween Pumpkin is not only a delicious food that is used for decorating the walkways during Halloween, it is power packed with nutrients that can benefit the skin immensely.

Oatmeal gently remove impurities from blocked pores and is an excellent remedy to treat dry skin. The honey will rehydrate and moisturize. Yogurt and honey both are superior anti-aging ingredients.

Yogurt improves the skin's elastin and will leave it bright and clear and helps to improve dark circles.

1.Add 1/4 cup oatmeal to a container

2.Add a small handful of diced sliced or chopped pumpkin in the container.

3.Add one large spoon of honey

4.Add one large spoon of plain yogurt

add a bit of warm water and blend into a paste.

You can thicken or weaken your mask by adding a

bit of warm water or adding more of an ingredient.

Was face clean and apply for 15 to 30 minutes wash with Luke warm water.

Enjoy your plump youthful beautiful hydrated skin!

Melon honey egg white, cornmeal yogurt

This is a mask scrub.

Melon is one of the earliest and first fruit to be made popular. They are from the bronze

age 1350 and 1120bc and is a low calorie food that is packed with nutrients and carotenoids

Anti-oxidants vitamin c and A and other minerals. Melons are rejuvenating and will revitalize tired skin. Honey moisturises and tightens pores and is a great rejuvenator. Yogurt improves the skin's elastin and will leave it bright and clear and helps to improve dark circles.

Cornmeal with its zinc manganese iron and copper and trace minerals gently scrubs away dead skin, and eggs are full of protein.

1.Add a small handful of diced or sliced yellow or red melon in a container.

2.Add two large spoon full of cornmeal

3.Add 1/4 cup of plain yogurt

4.Add three large spoon of honey

5.white of an egg

Blend crush mix together until smoothly blend. You can thicken or weaken your mask by adding a bit of warm water or adding more of an ingredient.

Wash face clean and apply for 15 to 30 minutes wash with Luke warm water or remove with warm cloth. Enjoy clean smooth soft and beautiful skin!

Quick Note

Any leftover mask can be stored in the refrigerator but make sure to use within a week. The sugar and oil mask can be stored a bit longer like two to three weeks.

About The Author

I am a supporter of green and organic heathy living. I tried to promote healthy
lifestyle choices whichever way I can.